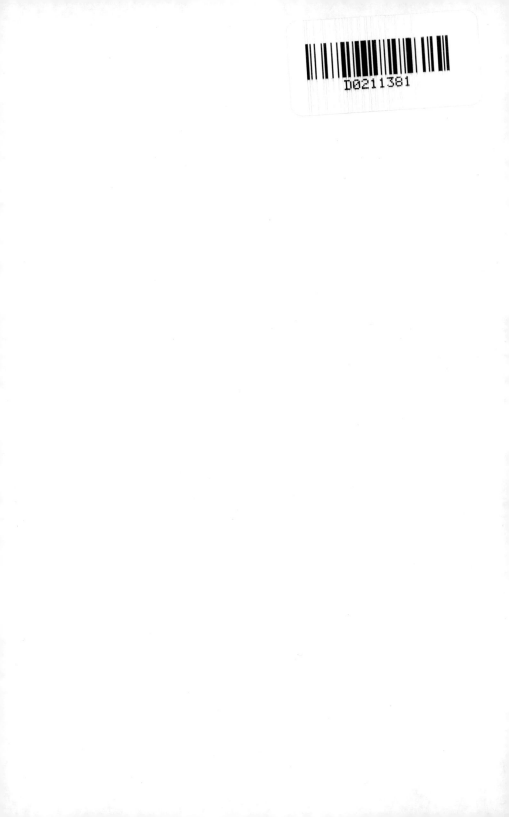

KISS
YOUR LIFE
HELLO

Health and Recovery with PSP

By Dr. Howard Peiper

ISBN 0-9702964-7-9
Library of Congress Catalog Card Number 2003106178
Printed in USA

Kiss Your Life Hello is not intended as medical advice, but as suggested complementary therapeutic regimens, to be considered only if deemed adequate by both patients and their chosen health professional. It is written solely for informational and educational purposes.

ATN Publishing
561 Shunpike Rd.
Sheffield, MA 01257
413-229-7935

Table of Contents

Dedication

This book is dedicated to a Higher Source who ultimately inspires those scientists, beknown to them or not, to work hard and be thorough in their research. These gifted men and women have been able to harness the incredible healing power of PSP. I am very grateful that my path has crossed with a wonderful human being, named Russ Hall. I thank him for introducing me to a product that is changing many lives. I believe in my heart that Russ and I together can change even more lives.

Introduction

Sit down before a fact as a little child,
be prepared to give up every preconceived notion,
follow humbly wherever and to whatever abysses nature
leads, or you shall learn nothing.
- Thomas Huxley

Nature and science are not always a marriage made in heaven. Until those in the health care profession realize the necessity of a bond between the two, millions of people will continue to suffer and die needlessly. This book is devoted to the benefits of what I believe to be the most powerful of whole food complexes.

It has been said, "The answers to all of man's medical questions and the cures for all ills have been placed on this earth by God. It is just up to us to find them." While this statement might have fallen on deaf ears up to a few years ago, it certainly rings true today. The cultural priorities of technology, progress, and seeking wealth have blinded us from seeing the truth: *To destroy our planet is to destroy the human race.* Coping with water and air pollution, making poor food choices, and entertaining unhealthy lifestyle options may be our sad but inevitable epitaph.

From the common cold to cancer we have become victims of free radicals, which ultimately wear down our immune system and inhibit its ability to defend and heal our body. These destructive culprits are found everywhere. They originate in food additives, byproducts of plastics, pollution, emotional stress and even sunlight. These unstable oxygen molecules are thought to be largely responsible for the degenerative processes that promote aging and even more importantly, are thought to be the largest contributor of disease. Research has proven that free radicals destroy. We subject ourselves to these killers, sometimes knowingly, but still we shake our heads and wonder why we develop disease.

What chance do we have against this villain? How do we eliminate these sources of destructive molecules? Improving air quality, purifying water, and improving diet does help. Reducing stress is easier said than done. Even if we attempt to change our lifestyles, we still may fall short of restoring our bodies to good health. Therefore, we must search for other means of combating free radical degeneration. The conventional weapons, called "antioxidants" are not enough.

While physicians have studied and trained hard to make a difference in peoples' lives, modern medicine often fails to achieve total wellness. Allopathic (traditional) medicines have been no match for many life-threatening diseases. Normal cells of the body can mutate into cancer cells and short circuit the immune system. This is possibly mediated by viruses, which may cause the body's defenses to attack themselves. These events have been implicated in diseases such as multiple sclerosis, possibly related to free radical damage. In effect we have become victims, a condition most likely brought about through our own short-sidedness and irresponsibility. Succumbing to our fast-paced lifestyles can result in ever increasing mortality numbers from heart disease, cancer, stroke, and conditions such as high blood pressure, high cholesterol, and diabetes. Is our society creating sufficient awareness of these problems to effectively address them or are we simply too busy trying to survive each day?

Needless to say, the preceding declaration of doom is quite depressing, but all is not lost. The outlook is no longer as hopeless as it once was. In the pages that follow, you will learn of a unique natural food formula unlike any other. It has been widely used for many years in Asia by doctors and other health care providers. It is made from a form of a *whole food complex* that is able to win the battle against free radical destruction—Polysaccharidepeptides, or PSP.

Results obtained from its users reveal that PSP can prevent disease, stave off degenerative processes and strengthen the immune system. When ingested PSP can assist the body in healing *at the cellular level*. As a form of a whole-food complex, PSP facilitates the body in taking an active role in healing and impacting the many conditions mediated by the derailment of the immune system. As the pages that follow will show, nature and science have joined together and harnessed PSP. Together they are truly creating miracles.

- *Dr. Howard Peiper*

Foreword

"Though this is a small book, the information it contains is gigantic. Valuable information offered by Howard Peiper touches the most important aspects of your health. Enjoy your reading experience, through which your life may be enriched. The information provided will allow you to be better prepared to make choices regarding the control of your health.

It is time for a paradigm shift. Our health system is in crisis. The relationship between patients and doctors has been compromised in the name of a third party liability or insurance. Physicians seem to rely on chemicals (pills) to suppress symptoms, schedule too little time for a comprehensive diagnosis, and are focused on wealth accumulation. These conditions can create confusing scenarios.

Many doctors have little knowledge that minor complaints or symptoms may be caused by an imbalance in the body, a lack of nutrients, or a build up of toxins. Their solution is to administer symptom-suppressing pills that may calm but rarely cure. Diagnoses, either real or created, are levied for various reasons as being part of the standard medical practice. In doing this, the opportunity of reaching the core of the problem and bringing corrective measures is lost. All this is done under the influence of fear. The patient is fearful of the diagnosis and the doctor is fearful of being wrong, most likely because of potential malpractice claims. Yet, fear is not conducive to healing.

I believe every doctor needs to read this book in order to better understand what alternatives may be available to prescription drugs that continue to silence symptoms without treating the cause. There are many alternatives such as analyzing the patient's acid/alkaline pH, a simple procedure that can offer much information. But yet, this is still far from being incorporated in the evaluation of the patient. Are we looking at the nutritional status of patients? Are we concerned with his or her antioxidant levels? What system of detoxification (ridding the body of toxins) is or could be safely implemented?

This book is a wake up call. It's time to take control. A doctor's primary responsibility is to the patient, not the insurance or drug company. Reading this book should be an event that is transformational for the patient. Dr. Peiper has given vital and cutting-edge information in a simple format. It is easy to assimilate and incorporate into your choice for protocols when dealing with ill health. It is refreshing to know there is a book that helps the patient relate symptoms to illness and one that offers an alternative to prescriptions that simply suppress those symptoms.

This book is extremely informative. All my patients will be invited to feast on it and I will make every effort to bring it to as many colleagues as time will permit. It is rewarding to know that there are writers taking the necessary steps to bring sound information to today's society. Howard, I am grateful for your research. May the good Lord give you His many blessings.
-*Esteban Genao, MD, FAAP*

Chapter One

Origin and Function

Rice is the culinary culture as well the basis for economical solvency in many societies. For example, the Burmese cultural history embraces ancient folklore where the Kachins people of northern Myanmar were sent forth from the center of the Earth with seeds of rice. These people were directed to a wondrous country where everything was perfect and where rice grew well. Today rice remains as their leading crop and a most revered food. In Bali, it is believed that the Lord Vishnu caused the Earth to give birth to rice, and the God Indra taught the people how to raise it. In both myths rice is considered a gift of the gods. Even in modern times the people of both countries treat rice with according reverence and its cultivation is tied to elaborate rituals.

By contrast, a Thai myth tells of rice being a gift of animals rather than of gods. This was a time when Thailand had been engulfed by severe weather and wracked with floods. After the land finally drained, people came down from the hills where they had taken refuge only to discover that all the plants had been destroyed and there was little to eat. They survived through hunting although animals were scarce. According to the writings, one day the people saw a dog coming across a field, and hanging on the dog's tail were bunches of long, yellow

1

seeds. They planted these seeds. Rice grew, and hunger disappeared. Throughout Thailand today, tradition holds that "the precious things are not pearls and jade but are the five grains," of which rice is the first. While most modern Thai's may intellectually dismiss its supernatural role, they cannot deny the enormous cultural importance of rice in their country, and also in most of the other rice-producing and rice-consuming countries of the world.

Science Meets Myth

Scientists have utilized ancient Thai folk medicine, techniques, and theory, combined with modern and sophisticated technology to produce polysaccharidepeptides or PSP. Alphaglycanology is a proprietary and innovative process employing biotechnology and nanotechnology. The purpose of the Alphaglycanology technique is to mechanically hydrolyze polysaccharides[1] and polypeptides[2] in cereal grains, from specially selected fractions of rice grains, harvested at the proper age. The grain is grown in an area where the soils are alkaline in nature and continuously enriched with natural organic matter containing abundant spirulina[3] found in the water. The rice is organically grown, free of pesticides and insecticides and is not modified in any way.

By bonding the polysaccharidepeptides together under controlled humidity, temperature and pressure, a naturally hydrolyzed alpha-glycan is formed. Therefore, when PSP enters the body, the cells can recognize it as a biological fuel for utilization by the mitochondria for the production of the cellular energy or *ATP* (adenosine triphosphate).

The special characteristics of PSP, produced with the Alphaglycanology process, allows for 100 percent

---

[1] any of the more complex carbohydrates
[2] molecular chain of amino acids
[3] a superior source of essential nutrients and antioxidants

bioavailability.[4] When consumed, these unique functional genomic nutrients are readily assimilated facilitating an improvement of the intracellular environment. This is essential for DNA repair and the resulting enhanced gene expression. Correspondingly, the environment manifested in the body is vitally essential for optimal health. The alphaglycanology process employed by scientists to produce PSP has shown its ability to effectively preserve the functional value of the phytonutrients.[5]

Scientists have found that when certain species of rice grains are grown under optimal conditions, and are harvested at the proper age, they contain top quality functional and essential nutrients such as specific polysaccharides, polypeptides, the amino acids, vitamins, minerals, and antioxidants (gamma oryzanol, tocopherol tocotrienols). Rice grains meeting these criteria are perfectly suited to enhance the cellular energy (ATP) production of the mitochondria for DNA repair and cellular regeneration. They can combat free radicals and enhance the detoxification process establishing an anabolic (building) phase so that the body's natural healing power may function optimally. The unique combination of these antioxidants, organic mineral amino acid compounds, and polysaccharides, has the ability to stimulate the body to naturally regulate a state of *homeostasis* (when the body is in balance). This results in balanced levels of blood sugar, cholesterol, triglycerides, blood pressure, body temperature, electrolytes, and pH.

pH Balance
The scale used to measure the body's acidity and alkalinity is called pH, normally measured in a range from one to fourteen. A neutral solution, neither acidic nor alkaline, has a pH of seven; acid is less than seven, alkaline is more

---

[4] total absorption on a cellular level
[5] Patented by Macro Food Tech Co., LTD Thailand.

than seven. The blood must be kept within the very narrow range of pH 7.4 to maintain homeostasis (balance).

Unfortunately, the average North American diet is very high in acid foods, such as sugar, refined carbohydrates and starch. These are not conducive to maintaining proper pH balance in the body and raise acid levels. To prevent disease from getting a foothold in this acid environment it is imperative that homeostasis be restored, which can be accomplished by adding trace minerals to the diet. This acidic condition is caused by metabolic waste. When trace minerals are in sufficient quantity they bind with the waste and flush it out through the urine thus returning the body to a more balanced state.

Excessive acid waste literally attacks the joints, tissues, muscles, organs, and glands, causing minor to major dysfunction. If it affects the joints, arthritis may develop; affects on the muscles may result in myofibrosis (aching muscles); attacks on the organs and glands, can cause a myriad of illnesses. The more acidic the body is, the more compromised the immune system becomes. A constant diet of foods excessively high in protein and sugar results in a more acidic body and weakens the immune system allowing conditions like chronic fatigue syndrome, cancer, MS, and arthritis to gain a foothold.

pH-balancing the body slightly more on the alkaline side than on the acid should be a daily goal. Because PSP is made from a whole food that is grown in an alkalized, mineral-enriched environment, it has the ability to facilitate a slightly alkaline pH balance. When the pH is balanced in the body, it is able to totally absorb all nutrients from foods and supplements. PSP efficiently creates and maintains a pH-balanced body.

Detoxification

An important function of PSP is its ability to detoxify[6] the body. Avoiding contact with toxins on a daily basis is virtually impossible, and a buildup of these toxins within the body results in many forms of illness. Cleanliness, externally and internally, is essential to good health. PSP assists this process because it works on the entire body to remove toxins from the system. When these toxins are eliminated PSP helps support and strengthen the glandular system helping the body heal itself.

The colon and the bowel become the depository for all waste material after food nutrients are extracted into the bloodstream. Decaying food ferments and forms gases as well as second and even third generation toxins. Thus the colon becomes a breeding ground for putrefactive bacteria, viruses, parasites, yeast and more. Because of PSP's fiber-like structure the peristalsis movement of the colon is strengthened and bowel movements are healthier and more regular, better facilitating the elimination process. Healthy intestines are the body's second immune system. Therefore, it is essential to keep them free of putrefied waste.

---

[6] to remove a poison or toxin

Chapter Two

The Immune System

No illness which can be treated by diet should be treated by any other means.
–Moses Maimonides, the great physician of 12th century

The immune system's basic function is to protect us against infection, illness and disease of all kinds. It fights off thousands of predatory environmental and infectious microorganisms, which can invade and damage virtually every part of the body. The immune system has the ability to expel pathogens (virus' bacteria, etc.), toxic chemicals, and tumorous cells that are generated through mutation. It also aids the body in tissue repair and healing and strives to maintain homeostasis (balance) in the body.

The immune system involves a finely tuned, highly integrated series of events that destroy a would-be invader. Once the immune system identifies an unwanted guest, it brings an awesome array of chemical and cellular weapons to banish the perpetrators. This non-specific, intricate, and elaborate immune response can readily discriminate between the "self" and "non-self", that is, cells that are a normal part of the body versus alien organisms. The innate intelligence of the immune system insures that the body does not turn on itself and lose the ability to distinguish between the "good and bad" cells.

Autoimmunity

When the immune system loses the ability to distinguish between self and nonself it may develop an autoimmunity (the body manufacturing antibodies and T-cells directed against its own cells, cell components or even specific organs). Autoimmune responses include allergies, asthma, rheumatoid arthritis, dermatitis, diabetes, systemic lupus erythematosis, multiple sclerosis, fibromyalgia and also may be the underlying factor in numerous chronic conditions. When the body is under constant exposure to various pathogens the immune system will become over stimulated resulting in autoimmunity.

Weakened Immunity

When the immune system is working properly we remain healthy. However, the immune system can and does become compromised. This may be a result of the following: incessant environmental assault such as from exposure to pseudo-estrogens; pesticides and pollutants in air, food and water; certain medications; persistent metabolic damage, (for example, high free-radical stress); poor nutrition, chronic infection or advancing age; and strenuous physical activity and emotional stress. As you can see, numerous diverse factors may compromise the immune system and disturb its exquisitely balanced components.

It is no secret that our body is put under physical and emotional stress warding off the above-mentioned multi-faceted assaults. When our bodies become overwhelmed the regulatory features of the immune system weaken and become less effective resulting in: fatigue; loss of stamina and energy; frequent colds and infections; loss of appetite and weight loss; fever and night sweats; skin rashes and cold sores; diarrhea; increased severity of allergy symptoms; swollen lymph nodes, and other symptoms of immune deficiencies.

In time, these conditions can exacerbate the initial symptoms into more serious immuno-compromised conditions (such as chronic fatigue, cancer, HIV, etc.). It is widely believed that cancer may be caused by a decline in the immune system function attributed to aging, lifestyle and other factors. The AIDS virus is known to destroy our immune cells and trigger a multitude of bodily system breakdowns.

Over time, normal cell-mediated immunity may become inadequate or malfunction. This may allow multiple genetic mutations in the same location (malignant transformations) resulting in abnormal growth. The degenerative process is generally quite slow and elusive. It may take many years and many bouts of illness to truly manifest itself where a diagnosis is levied.

PSP has strong immune-stimulating properties. Health care practitioners have consistently observed the therapeutic benefits produced by polysaccharidepeptides (PSP) for a wide range of health problems. It has been shown to promote vast improvement in cases of many common but serious health problems, ranging from cancer, chronic fatigue syndrome, high blood pressure, rheumatoid arthritis, Parkinson's, Alzheimer's, diabetes, hepatitis, high cholesterol, tumors, Tourette's, irritable bowel syndrome.[7]

To maintain good health, minimize the frequency and severity of all illnesses, and recover quickly, it is imperative that the immune system function efficiently and optimally. The more hazards we expose the body to, the greater the call for the immune system to maintain our health. Natural immune support is very important, making dietary additions such as PSP a primary consideration.

---

[7] Ishak, Dr. Mohammed, "Possible Solutions to the Global Health Problems," *Nature's Journal*, April 2002.

Chapter Three

PSP and Anti-Aging

Aging—it's happening to everybody. Time is accelerating the aging process faster than we'd like. But, even though the hourglass tells us we're older the passage of time isn't really what ages us. The aging culprit is the process that creates a reduction of healthy cells in our body.

Cells don't age; they're sloughed off as their efficiency diminishes and are replaced by new ones. With proper nutrition cell restoration continues in excess of what is generally considered a normal life expectancy. Industrialized civilization breeds environmental pollutants, diets full of chemicals and additives, vitamin and mineral deficiencies, and the overuse of prescription drugs. This menu of assaults gives rise to an early retirement in the cemetery. Today, industrialized countries boast statistics that claim 80 percent of the population in excess of sixty-five years old is chronically ill, usually with arthritis, diabetes or high blood pressure.[8]

The key to long life is emotional and physical balance (homeostasis). Our general loss of vitality and disease originate from poor diet, life-style choices, or from

---

[8] Page, Linda, ND, PhD, *Healthy Healing 11th Edition*, Traditional Wisdom, 2000.

long-term environmental assaults. Yet, there is hope. Youthfulness is restored from the inside, by strengthening our lean body mass, metabolism, and immune response with good nutrition, regular exercise, fresh air, and a positive mental attitude.

Fountain of Youth

Through my research I have determined that PSP can play a big role in our search for the "fountain of youth." The antioxidant properties of PSP prevent body components from destruction by free radicals—a key to anti-aging.

The three important contributors to aging are: cell and tissue damage caused by free radicals;[9] reduced immune response, and enzyme depletion in the body due to diets composed of enzyme deficient foods (cooked or processed.)

Free radicals, (highly active compounds produced when molecules react with oxygen,) play a key role in the deterioration of the body. Under assault from chemicalized foods and environmental pollutants, our bodies generate excesses of these cell damagers. After years of free-radical assaults cells become irreplaceably lost from major organs such as the lungs, liver, kidneys, the brain, and particularly our nervous system. This loss is seen as a primary cause of aging.

Alzheimer's, Parkinson's, and Multiple Sclerosis are thought to be associated with the aging process due to three potent neurotoxins, Beta-Amyloid, Glutamate, and Peroxides, that can lead to nerve cell damage and destruction. These molecules disrupt and destroy normal nerve cell function.

Studies reveal that PSP has been shown to preserve nerve cell function by supplying food and nutrients at the cellular level. The concept is simple. Provide the

---

[9] unstable fragments of molecules produced from oxygen and fats in cells

cell with food easily recognized and utilized by the cell's DNA (the "molecule of life") to generate energy. This will provide the vehicle for repairing cell damage. This is incredible news for people with Alzheimer's and Creutzfeldt-Jakob diseases. Both illnesses manifest when a neurotoxin, called Beta Amyloid, deposits itself in the brain and disrupts communication between nerve cells. Scientists have tried to treat the diseases by attacking the protein deposits but to date this approach has not been successful.

A new study shows that by helping nerve cells produce normal proteins these connections can actually be rejuvenated.[10] In this study, nerve cells exposed to three of the most potent neurotoxins were ultimately protected from damage after adding PSP to the medium. A degree of cellular regeneration of the nerve dendrites and axons was also seen. These extraordinary results have consistently been observed in subsequent research.

Superoxide dismutase (SOD) is an extremely potent antioxidant enzyme that fights cellular damage from single oxygen molecules (also known as free radicals). As an enzyme, SOD has particular value helping to protect against cell destruction. Research suggests that SOD may be the most important enzyme in the body for the control of free radicals, keeping our cell membranes young, supple, and healthy (anti-aging). Although SOD has been sold as a supplement, research shows that oral SOD is destroyed by the digestive system before it can fight free radicals and repair damaged joints. This suggests that the most viable means of building healthy levels of SOD in the body would be to consume natural food substances that bind protein to SOD and therefore deliver it via the digestive system to the body, without being destroyed in

[10] Sawatsri, Sayan, MD, Yankunthong, Wanphen, M.Sc, *PSP may Prevent Neuron Vulnerablility in Human Neuroblastoma Cells,* PMK Research Institute, Bangkok, Thailand, March, 2001.

the gut. PSP facilitates that process and increases the level of SOD in the body.

There are numerous antioxidants[11] made by the body as well as antioxidants found through supplementation or in our diets. Nutrients like vitamins E and C, beta-carotene and the trace mineral selenium root out any free radicals that make it past the antioxidants enzymes. It is necessary to support the body's own production of antioxidant enzymes (SOD) because they remove free radicals three to ten times faster than the nutrient antioxidants. The body will benefit far more if it can produce its own antioxidant enzymes, and that is what PSP facilitates.

PSP is a premier agent for reversing the causes of aging by utilizing the following:
1. Increasing the level of SOD (superoxide dismutase), the master antioxidant;
2. Enhancing nucleotide production for DNA repair;
3. Enhancing cellular environment for improved genetic expression;
4. Increasing pro-enzyme and probiotic (friendly intestinal bacteria) activities.

"Since I started taking PSP my sexual performance has been enhanced. I am sixty-one years old, in a relationship with a 44-year-old female and was dismayed when I found my sexual energy diminishing. I had thought of taking *Viagra*. However, my Naturopathic Doctor suggested trying PSP. It worked and I am so grateful that I listened to him."
–Julio Cabral, Mexico City, Mexico

---

[11] a substance that inhibits oxidation or reactions promoted by oxygen or peroxides

"I took PSP for general maintenance and to my grateful surprise, I discovered that at least 50 percent of my face wrinkles have disappeared, and my skin tightened up. I have tried everything short of a surgical face-lift. I am happy to discover an alternative that works. This will be a youth-saver for all post-menopausal women (and men)!"
-Nina A., East Canaan, CT

Chapter Four

The Brain and Mental Function

The brain is a delicate and complex structure. As the control center of all physical and intellectual activity in the body it utilizes as many as 100 billion different cells, with millions and millions of neurons forming a seemingly innumerable number of connections. It is responsible for all of our internal functions and our interactions with our external surroundings. In order to maintain this relationship, the brain must be functioning properly. For us to enjoy life to the fullest, we need to be in control. Optimal functioning is desired for optimal interaction. Around the age of thirty, neurons (brain cells) begin to die (or go dormant). After this age, they die at a faster rate than they are replaced, thus beginning the degenerative process that becomes more and more obvious as we get older.

Neurons are large cells, which require large amounts of energy and proper nutrition to function normally. The brain receives 15-20 percent of the body's total blood supply and uses 15-20 percent of the body's total inhaled oxygen, which along with glucose, is used by the brain to produce and use 15-20 percent of the body's total ATP (adenosine triphosphate) energy. Unlike most other cells, which can burn fat or glucose for their energy needs, neurons can only burn glucose. Under normal conditions our brain cells typically consume 50

14

percent of the total blood glucose. Therefore, neurons and cells in the brain are dependent upon a continuous and uninterrupted rich blood supply to maintain normal energy metabolism and avoid cellular injury or death.

Under normal conditions, with adequate oxygen supply, these neurons convert glucose into (ATP) for three reasons:

1. Cell maintenance: Since neurons don't reproduce and must last a lifetime, they are continually expending energy to repair or replace various cell parts—cell membrane segments, microtubules, mitochondria, etc.

2. Neurotransmitter operation: Neurons use ATP to produce, transport, package, secrete, and reuptake neurotransmitters such as acetylcholine and serotonin, which provide vital cell-to-cell communication.

3. Electrical energy: Huge amounts of ATP are necessary to facilitate the frequent discharges of electrical energy from the neuron through the cell body to the transmitting end—the axon. For this electrical process to occur there must be a rapid and continuous exchange of sodium and potassium ions back and forth across the neuronal membranes.

Over a lifetime, there can be slow and subtle memory loss resulting from brain-energy losses due to cerebral arteriosclerosis, ministrokes, neurotoxins (glutamate, beta-amyloid, and peroxides), or brief interruptions of brain oxygen supply (often caused by blood vessel spasm). In addition to memory impairment, this brain energy crisis may also cause occasional confusion or lapses in concentration, and learning difficulties.

For reasons we are only beginning understand, the neuron-replacement process is far more evident in some people than in others. One octogenarian will be fully self sufficient, remembering not only what they need to do for that day, but also the details of some event that happened over forty years ago. However, others may not remember their own telephone number or the names of their children or grandchildren.

At a more advanced stage the brain energy crisis may show itself as senility or senile dementia, and eventually may terminate in coma or death. The severity of dementia is directly correlated to the loss of functional brain tissue independent of the primary neuropathology. If someone's brain is not working correctly it is largely because of brain disease (such as Alzheimer's, Parkinson's, brain tumor, infection, vascular disturbances), injury (such as from brain trauma, stroke, stress, neurotoxins, alcohol or drugs), or deficiencies of EFA's (essential fatty acids) or B complex vitamins.

Symptoms of Cognitive Deterioration
Cognitive deterioration can involve the loss or decline of any of the cognitive functions including:

- Memory
- Orientation
- Information fixation
- Judgment
- Attention
- Perception

Major contributing factors to cognitive degeneration may include the following:

- Chronic circulatory problems in the brain: This includes a variety of medical conditions that decrease the delivery of blood flow to the brain reducing glucose, oxygen, and nutrients to the brain cells;
- Various cerebral disorders: These include Alzheimer's or Parkinson's diseases;
- Cerebral hemorrhage;

- Transient ischaemic attacks (TIA): an inter-
rupted blood flow to the brain;
- Various brain-toxic substances: We cite ex-
amples such as alcohol, opiates, (morphine, her-
oin), cocaine, amphetamines, hallucinogens, (STP,
LSD, marijuana, etc.) and neurotoxins (glutamate,
beta-amyloid and peroxides);
- Various prescribed medications: These may be
very toxic to the brain and may cause memory loss, confusion or depression, and may have an adverse effect on
brain function. Various prescription medications can include: pain killers, antidepressants, tranquilizers, sleeping
pills, antihistamines, corticosteroids, heart and blood
pressure medication.

Individuals with vascular disease or dementia attributed to Alzheimer's often have a disturbance in antioxidant balance that may predispose one to increased oxidative stress. This would then be a potential therapeutic
area for antioxidant supplementation.

Enhanced memory function
PSP is recommended for cerebral circulatory disorders
such as memory problems, acute stroke, aphasia (loss of
the power of expression), apraxia (inability to coordinate
movements), motor disorders, dizziness and other cere-
bro-vestibular (inner-ear) problems, and headache. PSP
can often be beneficial for acute or chronic ophthalmo-
logic diseases of various origins, and may improve vision.
PSP also has a very powerful stimulating effect on memory because of its effect on the brain's metabolism.

PSP increases the metabolism in the brain several ways:
- It increases the rate at which brain cells produce ATP (which is the cell molecule that creates energy);

- It speeds up the use of glucose in the brain;
- It speeds up the use of oxygen in the brain.

The result is that the cells of the brain can better retain information causing the individual to remember more. PSP has been reported as showing promising benefits for the following conditions:

stroke	depression
vertigo	tinnitus
Meniere's Syndrome	migraine headaches
sleep disorders	macular degeneration
mood changes	convulsions
Tourette's Syndrome	Multiple Sclerosis
ADD/ADHD	Cerebral Palsy

PSP Increases Neurotransmitters

PSP stimulates cognitive enhancement primarily through its influence on important neurotransmitters. These neurotransmitters relay information between neurons and rely on specialized brain chemicals to function properly. While memory is an extremely complex phenomenon, neuronal transmission is even more complex. There are more than one hundred different neurotransmitters that have been identified.

Depressed levels of certain neurotransmitters are associated with psychiatric disorders. Depression has been linked with depressed levels of serotonin and Parkinson's has been linked with depressed levels of dopamine. An overabundance of dopamine is associated with Tourette's syndrome (an involuntary movement and vocal disorder, often socially disabling).

Neurotransmitters are responsible for the transmission of information between neurons, indicating that they are necessary for *all* cognitive functions.

PSP supports neuronal transmission by:

- increasing levels of noradrenaline (thinking, learning planning);
- balancing levels of dopamine (libido, information processing);
- increasing levels of acetylcholine (memory);
- increasing levels of serotonin (mood, sleep, balances appetite, lowers substance cravings).

Please take note that depression is a symptom of insufficient serotonin levels, which is often caused by prolonged exposure to stressors. Scientists have found that a positive therapeutic effect of PSP was shown in patients who exhibited pronounced depressive states of varied origins. In a recent study, a substantial decrease or complete disappearance of the clinical manifestation of depression was noted in 65 percent of the patients. Serotonin has the ability to help the body adapt to stress. PSP can raise serotonin levels thereby helping the body resist chronic stress and mood disorders related to low levels of serotonin.

"I cannot say enough good things about this miraculous food. For nine years I had suffered from Multiple Sclerosis experiencing vision problems, muscle weakness, fatigue, dizziness, and burning sensations in my feet. After taking PSP three times a day for several months, all of my symptoms disappeared. I am able to walk without a limp and climb stairs without the aid of a railing. I feel like I have truly found a miracle in my life."
-*Paula Barnes, Washington State*

Chapter Five

PSP and Diabetes

America is in the midst of a growing epidemic that now affects more than 18 million people. The medical pharmaceutical industry calls this metabolic disorder "diabetes" which occurs when the body is unable to properly utilize insulin, which is designed to help regulate glucose or blood sugar levels in the body. If blood sugar concentrations rise a number of critical body functions are affected such as metabolism, fluid retention, blood-sugar regulation and liver function. When the body produces too much insulin and loses its ability to respond appropriately a condition develops known as insulin resistance syndrome. It is estimated that nearly 80 million Americans have this problem, and most of them don't even know it.

PSP works at the cellular and molecular level providing each and every cell with the energy it needs to metabolize glucose, rid the body of toxins and waste products, and begin cellular regeneration. The molecular structure of PSP allows for improved absorption and assimilation of glucose through direct absorption into the cell. The properties in PSP help keep the glucose-energy metabolism system finely tuned. This dramatically decreases the workload of the liver by enhancing direct cellular absorption of glucose, reducing the amount of insulin release and therefore decreasing the risk of other metabolic disorders.

PSP will improve health conditions linked with diabetes. For example, one may experience:

- better balance of blood glucose;
- reduced fatigue and more energy;
- enhanced natural production of antioxidants to reduce free radical damage;
- less damage to glucose/energy metabolism;
- better healing of diabetic gangrene, greatly reducing the risk of amputation.

"L.H., age sixty-nine, is amazed that he can walk from his bed to the bathroom without excruciating pain. Since being diagnosed Type II Diabetic in 1993, L.H. has suffered burning and painful tingling sensations in his toes and feet. He experienced such pain that he couldn't bear to walk even the short distance to the bathroom without something on his feet. Like most of us L.H. was very skeptical of the restorative properties of PSP. The pain in his feet and the daily annoyance of taking up to five pills to control his blood sugar prompted him to give PSP a try. Is he ever glad he did! After just three weeks of taking only one scoop a day in the morning, L.H. has cut out his medication by 75 percent. Not only has his blood sugar stabilized, he now has enough energy to go to the gym. Perhaps best of all, he walks with much less pain than before taking PSP." -*Tien Huynh, New Orleans, LA*

"I've had serious health problems during the last ten years, including Type II Diabetes and colds that would develop into walking pneumonia. Allergic reactions to antibiotics made it all the more difficult to control the illnesses. At the beginning of 2003 I was told about a new whole food supplement called PSP which I began taking in a cup of green tea.

I have had circulation problems for years and although the condition has improved, my feet were still numb and cold to the touch. My remedy for this was to apply *Vicks Vapor Rub* on my feet and wear socks to keep them warm. It helped, but didn't solve the problem. I was quite surprised at what happened on the second day of using PSP when I realized that I had forgotten to use the *Vicks*. My feet started itching and I couldn't stop moving my toes and rubbing my feet together. It was evident that the circulation was returning to my feet and they were healing! I was excited because I feared my circulation problems might lead to serious complications, common in diabetics.

After reporting my newfound 'cure' to my doctor in Las Colinas, he said that he would monitor my progress and reduce my medication if needed. I checked my blood pressure and blood glucose twice a day and noticed that my blood pressure had dropped the first day I took PSP. The average for the last two weeks was 122/68 (had previously tested at 131/88) and my blood glucose average for two weeks was 111 and had been 128. When I was first diagnosed with Type II Diabetes there were times when my eyesight would blur and I was unable to focus. After taking PSP, I find I rarely use glasses now for reading or writing.

I had been on PSP for six weeks and noticed many changes. I was now free of rashes from allergies. The brown spots on my arms and hands were fading, my eyebrows were growing thicker and there was a marked improvement in my digestion. My metabolism must have increased because I lost inches. My break through came during the second week after I began taking PSP. I often use a full-body vibrator with heat and never felt the vibration in my ankles and feet until now. I now also find that my energy is unbelievably strong."
-*Donna Marshall, Grand Prairie, TX*

Chapter Six

PSP for High Cholesterol
and Cardiovascular Disease

According to recent data, over 36 million Americans have a total serum cholesterol count of over 240, which puts them at risk for coronary heart and cardiovascular disease (heart attacks, angina,). Coronary heart disease refers to heart damage that occurs when the coronary arteries become blocked or narrowed due to a buildup of plaque or oxidized cholesterol. For men and women whose cholesterol count falls in the range of 200-240, as it does for over 54 million people, the risk of heart disease is double that of those individuals whose cholesterol levels indicate below 200.

Genetic predisposition and the measured ratio of LDL cholesterol to HDL may determine who will develop coronary disease. However, high total cholesterol is considered a major indicator of potential cardiovascular disease, and can also contribute to gallstones, impotence, mental impairment and hypertension. Even more serious is the risk for cholesterol buildup to break off and lodge in the heart or the brain causing heart attack or stroke.

A study performed at Cho-ray hospital in Vietnam was conducted with three hundred doctors and nurses who have experienced some type of heart condition.[12] They participated in a ninety-day test in which they supplemented their diets with PSP on a daily basis. The results were astonishing. Within the test period, 100 percent of the subjects showed significant improvement in their heart conditions. They are now administering PSP to all of their intensive care unit patients.

This study revealed that PSP had a powerful effect on cellular function, which produced:

- lower LDL cholesterol;
- increased HDL cholesterol;
- decreased hypertension;
- reduced apolipoprotein-B (complexes of fat and protein found in blood plasma);
- better ratio of LDL to HDL;
- lower risk of heart attack.

Terry Johnson, from Michigan, had a high cholesterol level and was unable to take the vast amount of conventional medications prescribed for her. She was introduced to PSP and gave this report. "After taking PSP for six weeks, my cholesterol level dropped from 318 to 225. My doctor was very pleased and advised that I should continue taking it."

---

[12] Cho-Ray Hospital in Hanoi, Vietnam, Study conducted by J.Toan, MD, March 2003.

Chapter Seven

PSP and Cancer

Cancer high-risk groups are generally linked to genetics and age, although stress is currently being considered a contributor because it weakens the immune system and makes the body less likely to control cancer cell growth. Cancer is the abnormal growth of cells in the body. It is a result of normal cell mutation through its genetic chromosome material, RNA and DNA. Normally cells replicate themselves continually at a rate synchronous with normal growth and repair in a manner specific for its purpose in the body. Cancerous cells multiply faster than normal and lose normal differentiation sometimes forgetting to die.

Chemical and environmental factors may be responsible for 90 percent of all cancers. Elevated risk of cancer from hormone imbalances and toxic buildup in the cells, especially in the colon, can actually be linked to environmental assaults from pesticides and meat hormone residues. While cancer is one of the leading causes of death today, many types of cancer are preventable.

To keep cancer from compromising the body we must strengthen the immune system by naturally enhancing the cellular rejuvenation process. PSP can be a facilitator of this process. As the body's cells become healthier, they will stimulate the immune system and improve its functionality. Also, because PSP balances the pH in the body, the oxygen level is raised. Since cancer *cannot* live in a highly oxygenated environment its survival will be compromised.

Some aggressive forms of cancer treatment often are exceedingly stressful to the body. Side effects can be debilitating, for example, hair loss and the "wasting disease" associated with chemotherapy. Patients using PSP have shown a reduction in the severity of these side effects. Used in conjunction with conventional therapy, PSP can strengthen the immune function and provide a more therapeutic platform for recovery.

"I am forty-nine years old have had rheumatoid arthritis. I have been in the UCLA experimental program on and off for many years, taking a prescription drug to control the pain. I am also afflicted with receding gums and I visit my dentist every three months to have him check on my condition.

One day when I was taking a shower I noticed there was a small lump on my neck. The fear of cancer immediately crossed my mind. The next day I saw my doctor and he told me to have an ultrasound and x-ray on my throat. I was right it was cancer.

My uncle had been using PSP and suggested it to me. Most of the people know that I am skeptical about new products but, at this point, I had nothing to lose. During my check-up one month later, my doctor was surprised that the lump had completely disappeared and advised that I continue taking the PSP since it seemed to be helping my condition. By the way, my gums are less painful and I am not as tired as I used to be. PSP has helped me at just the right time." *-Linda Arnold, Los Angeles, CA*

"I've been taking PSP for a month on the advice of my naturopathic doctor. Prior to taking PSP, I had just quit chemotherapy treatments and my body was greatly

debilitated from its side effects. I started a new regimen, which included PSP and noticed that my mood, energy and feeling of well-being has returned. Today I am feeling as good as I felt before contracting cancer. I had a second surgery for an incisional hernia repair and within two days I was walking my usual three miles. My surgical scar has also completely healed. As an RN, I know that this rapid a recovery is quite unusual and I have attributed it to the PSP and following my doctor's other suggestions on healthy living. I'm confident that this regime will help me to continue being strong and cancer free."
-Barbara Bankey, Albuquerque, NM

Chapter Eight

PSP and Chronic Fatigue Syndrome (CFS)

By giving the body the right nutrition,
most diseases would be eradicated.
–Dr. Linus Pauling, Winner of two Nobel Prizes

Most researchers believe that Chronic Fatigue Syndrome (CFS) is a result of mixed infections with several pathogens such as environmental pollutants and chemical contaminants. These contribute to CFS by reducing our immune response, thereby allowing the syndrome to develop. In addition, growing evidence points to the fact that exhausted adrenal glands from high stress lifestyles and an imbalance in the hypothalamic-pituitary-adrenal axis can exacerbate the illness. CFS is a response (or lack of immune response) to the ever-increasing mental, emotional and physical stressors in our environment. As our body's immunity drops lower and lower almost any disruption in our health or emotional state can be the final trigger for Chronic Fatigue Syndrome.[13]

Research indicates PSP can help balance immune system functions in two ways and therefore guard against CFS. PSP can directly and specifically stimulate the immune system by increasing the body's resistance to toxins

---

[13] Fibromyalgia, Lupus, Epstein-Barr virus, and Lyme disease share many symptoms with CFS.

that may accumulate during the development of infection when the immune system is first called into action. b) PSP helps to stabilize the hormone cortisol, which is responsible for how we respond to stress. Stress suppresses immunity and destroys our resistance to various forms of bacterial or viral attacks. When we are under stress, a great portion of the body's energy is expended. Chronic exposure to stress results in a lowered immune response and decreased health.

"Due to chronic fatigue traced to anemia, in 1999 I retired from being a very active office manager. I consulted with several medical doctors who were unable able to correct the situation. As time passed I became more fatigued and my blood pressure began to rise during exercise or stress. I was under constant medical attention without receiving any appreciable results. I was also diagnosed as being oxygen deprived (to the brain). In July, 2002, I became immobile and had to be placed on oxygen 100 percent of the time. If I removed the oxygen my skin became blue within minutes. In addition, my appetite disappeared and my stomach began to expand, similar to conditions seen in a starved child in Africa. I was for all practical purposes trapped in my living room by day and by night. I did not see any hope.

In December 2002 I was introduced to PSP. I took the recommended three scoops a day. On the third day I was able to go off the oxygen for a very short period of time and make breakfast for my husband for the first time in six months. On the fourth day I was able to go to the shopping mall and have my hair done (two hours without oxygen). On the fifth day I actually cleaned my house. During Christmas of 2002 my family celebrated what I considered to be a miracle.

On the first day of January 2003, only a month after I started taking PSP, I was relying on the oxygen only 5 percent of the time. My appetite was back to normal, my energy returned, and I felt like my old self. I believe that this product will extend my life for many years." -*Toni Garcia, Albuquerque, NM*

Chapter Nine

PSP and Hepatitis

The liver is an important organ involved in metabolizing toxins and medications to a less damaging substance. However, in its efforts to protect the body from harm the liver itself may become a victim of toxic exposure and be subject to hepatitis.

Hepatitis is a disease or condition marked by inflammation of the liver. There are several types of viral hepatitis: Type A is a viral infection passed through blood and feces; Type B is a sexually transmitted viral infection carried through blood, semen, saliva, and dirty needles; Type C is a post-transfusion form; and Type D is caused by the Epstein-Barr virus. All forms of hepatitis are characterized by the following conditions: fatigue; flu-like symptoms of exhaustion and diarrhea; enlarged, tender, congested, sluggish liver; loss of appetite to the point of anorexia; nausea; dark urine; gray stools; occasional vomiting; skin pallor and histamine itching; depression; skin jaundice; and cirrhosis of the liver.

Vaccinations are commonly prescribed for Hepatitis but natural therapies have also had overwhelming success in treating hepatitis cases, both in arresting viral replication, and in regeneration of the liver. PSP contains properties that can protect the liver from damage and even reverse damage that has already occurred. PSP works

31

against toxins and assaults that potentially damage the liver and has been found to help protect it from the detrimental effects of hepatitis.

Chapter Ten

PSP and Arthritis

Let thy food be thy medicine and
medicine be thy food.
–Hippocrates, the Father of Medicine

Normally considered to be an inevitable part of aging, some schools of thought deem the condition of arthritis to be a result of a toxic body trying to rid itself of waste. When salt combines with other wastes it precipitates out of the blood and lymph fluids, forming abrasive deposits. Ending up in the joints, these deposits may cause a condition known as bursitis and arthritis. Minerals normally carry these deposits out of the body. Our Western diets are deficient in the minerals needed by the body. This is due to over farming of the soil without mineral replacement. Foods grown in this manner (including both supermarket and organic varieties), are lacking the essential minerals needed by the body to function as designed.

Arthritis is one of the long-term effects of mineral imbalance and free radical damage. Mineral imbalance manifests as an acid condition in the body, and develops because our pH is not in homeostasis. With specific dietary changes, supplementation with PSP and a good mineral supplement, the pH can be better balanced resulting in arresting the pain and degeneration of even advanced arthritic conditions.

Because PSP is processed from specific rice grains that are grown in highly alkalized and mineralized soil, taking PSP daily will keep the pH of our body balanced. Cleansing and supporting the immune system will also help reduce the effects of arthritis.

"Be patient and PSP will astound you and bring you joy and happiness. I have learned that if it takes five years to get sick, it could take possibly five months to get well. PSP has made such a great difference in my overall health that I advise everyone to take PSP." With these words Jeff Thompson explains that PSP saved him from a long history of health problems, most significantly, severe arthritis, sinus and hay fever. Relief did not come overnight to Jeff. Indeed, everyone who takes PSP benefits at a different rate—some within hours or days, others weeks or months. Jeff fell into the latter category.

"My wife, Shamasi and I started taking PSP in the middle of January 2003. For years she had suffered from arthritis pain in both hands. By the end February her pain was gone. We both are experiencing wonderful results from taking PSP. I've had problems with ulcers and they are gone and what has really surprised me is that my Rosacea (red face) has almost disappeared. I am a true believer in this fantastic product."
-Jim and Shamsi McMahan, Sugar Land, TX

Chapter Eleven

Research and Studies[14]

PSP may prevent neuron vulnerability in human neuroblastoma cells (preliminary, unpublished data).
-*A study by Dean, M. Ishak, PhD,MD, College of Complementary Medicine, Malaysia*

Abstract (Preliminary data)

Objective: The current study investigated the neurotrophic and neuroprotective action of a unique formulation of Polysaccharidepeptides (PSP+), which consists of carbohydrate, crude protein, and essential minerals by using pressure and mechanical hydrolysis to make a complex formulation.
Methods: Using neuronal cell lines prepared from the LA-N-5 (Los Angeles Neuroblastoma) for Alzheimer's disease (AD) in complete media and treated with indicated manner, inverted microscopic evaluated morphological and biochemical analysis were conducted to determine the neurotrophic and neuroprotective properties of PSP+.
Results: Results of this analysis demonstrated that PSP+ significantly decreased neuronal cell death, a cellular

---

[14] The formulation used in the testing was a product labeled Vital PSP+

marker of memory formation. Dose response analysis (experiment going on) indicated that the lowest effective concentration of PSP+ exerted the minimal neurotrophic effect. Results of neuroprotection studies demonstrated that PSP+ induced highly significant neuroprotection against beta-amyloid, peroxides, and glutamate induced toxicity.

Discussion: Abnormality of glucose/energy metabolism shows relation to AD (1,2,2,4). PSP+ may prevent impairment of glucose/energy metabolism and may improve the ability of neurons to reduce the levels of free radicals (scavengers) and thereby affect ATP levels. (11,12).

Conclusion: PSP+ induced cellular markers of memory function in neurons critical to memory and vulnerable to negative effects of aging, cellular degeneration and Alzheimer's disease. Results of the current study could demonstrate the cellular mechanism of PSP+ on cognitive function and a possible intervention in Alzheimer's disease.

Key Words: Polysaccharidepeptides (PSP+), Cell Death, Alzheimer's disease (AD), Neuroprotective.

Control: Nerve cells

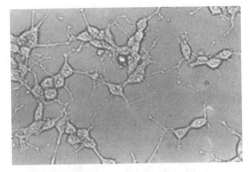

Same nerve cells injured by beta-amyloid neurotoxin.

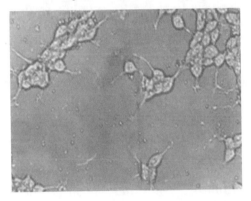

Same nerve cells rejuvenated
after being pretreated with PSP+

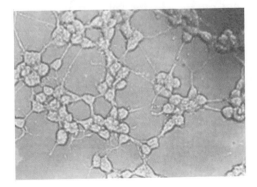

Introduction

1.1 Alzheimer's disease: A scientific mystery and major impact. Abnormality of glucose/energy metabolism shows relation to Alzheimer's disease (1,2,3,4). Degenerative and cell death are major causes in AD.

1.2 PSP+ is a complex formulation that consists of carbohydrate, crude protein and essential minerals by using pressure and mechanical hydrolysis to make a complex formulation designated PSP+(5).

1.3 PSP+ is very safe because it contains phytochemicals that have components of carbohydrates, crude protein and essential minerals by using pressure and mechanical hydrolysis to make a complex formulation designated PSP+. Evidence by observation from animal (pig) data showed that PSP+ could decrease morbidity from Ataxia (PSP+ may improve cerebral blood flow). In clinical use we found that PSP+ improves short and long term memory (6).

1.4 LA-N-5 (Neuroblastoma cell lines) have been used for model of Alzheimer's disease *in vitro* (7,8,9,10).

Objectives

1. To determine if PSP+ may promote neurotropic and neuroprotective actions that show decreased cell death (Apoptosis) in the Alzheimer model *in vitro*.

2. To determine if PSP+ shows neurotrophic and neuroprotective action in AD model and to determine what is the mechanism of PSP+.

For proposed mechanism of PSP+ induced neuroprotection in AD model *in vitro*.

Materials and Methods (1)

1. Neuronal culture

   Neuronal cells lines were prepared from the LA-N-5; Los Angeles Neuroblastoma derived from bone marrow metastasis of four-month-old male patient. Cells were propagated in RPMI 1640 supplemented with 10 percent FCS, 2mM glutamine, 50 IU/ml penicillin, 50 ug/ml streptomycin, and 1 ug/ml fungizone (complete medium).

2. Morphological analysis

   By using inverted microscopic evaluated morphological analysis of LA-N-5 in indicated conditions.

3. Neuronal

   Neuronal viability was determined by inclusion criteria of trypan blue.

4. The neurotrophic and neuroprotective action of PSP+ was determined by inducing other neurotoxic substrates as indicated conditions.

   1.1 Estrogen deprivation exposure: Neuronal viability was determined by estrogen deprivation exposure.

   1.2 Hydrogen peroxide exposure: 1uM $H2O2$ for 5 minutes at 37 deg. C. During exposure, E2 or PSP+ was added concurrently with $H2O2$. After 5 min. the culture was rinsed two times with HBS, and Fresh medium with E2 or PSP+ was replaced.

   1.3 Glutamate exposure: 0.2 uM Glutamate 20 min. at room temperature.

   1.4 Beta amyloid25-35 exposure: 8 ug/ml AB25-35 24. at 37 deg. C.

Results

* Neuroprotection by PSP+ against other neurotoxic results:

- o   Estrogen deprivation induced neurotoxicity
- o   Hydrogen peroxide induced neurotoxicity
- o   Glutamate induced neurotoxicity
- o   Beta amyloid25-35 induced neurotoxicity

* Dose dependent of PSP+ shows neuroprotection against other neurotoxins

Discussion

Abnormality of glucose/energy metabolism shows relation to AD (1,2,3,4). PSP+ may prevent impairment of glucose/energy metabolism and may improve the ability of neurons to reduce the levels of ("scavenger") free radicals and thereby affecting ATP levels (11,12).

Conclusions

- • PSP+ contains a unique formulation consisting of a complex form of carbohydrate, crude protein and essential minerals by using high pressure and mechanical hydrolysis to make a complex formulation designated polysaccharidepeptides (PSP+). PSP+, in vitro, has consistently demonstrated that it prevents cell death from other neurotoxicity agents.
- • PSP+ induced cellular markers of memory function in neurons critical to memory and vulnerable to negative effects of aging, cellular degeneration and Alzheimer's disease. Results of the current study could demonstrate the cellular mechanism of PSP+ on cognitive function and a possible intervention in Alzheimer's disease.

- In clinical application, PSP+ may promote cellular mechanism in memory and neuronal survival and may be used as a nutritional supplement in aging, cellular degenerative processes and a possible use for preventing Alzheimer's disease.

References

1. Blass, JP, Gibson, GE, Shimada, M, Kihara, T, Watanabe, M, and Kurinioto, K, (1980) "Brain carbohydrate metabolism and dementia," *Biochemistry of Dementia* (Burman, D. and Pennock, C.A., eds.), Wiley, London, pp 121-134.

2. Blass, JP, Sheu, KFR, and Cederbaum, JM, (1988), "Energy metabolism in disorders of the nervous system," *Rev. Neurol. (Paris),* 144, 543-563.

3. Beal, MF, (1992), "Does impairment of energy metabolism Result in excitotoxic neuronal death in neurodegenerative Diseases?" *Ann. Neurol.,* 31, 119-123.

4. Blass, JP, Sheu, KFR, and Tanzi, R, (1996), "a-Ketoglutarate dehydrogenase in Alzheimer's disease in Energy Metabolism," *Neurodgenerative Diseases (Fiskum, G, ed.),* Plenum, NY, pp. 185-192.

5. Laboratory report from Pacific Lab Services, Report No: /396-3971/LS/2001, Feb. 19th, 2001.

6. Interview with Medical Doctors Testimonial No.007, 018, 058 and 068.

7. Preuss, U, Mandelhow, EM, (1998) "Mitotic phosphorylation of tau protein in neuronal cell lines resembles phosphorylation in Alzheimer's disease." *Eur J Cell Biol,* 76 (3): 176-84.

8. Mesco, ER, Timiras, PS., "Tau-ubiquitin protein conjugates a human cell line," *Mech Ageing Dev* 199; 61 (1): 1-9.

9. Davis, PK, Johnson, GV, (1994) "Monoclonal antibody Alz-50 reacts with bovine and human ser albumin," *J Neurosci Res,;* 39(5): 589-94.

10. Fabrizi, C, Businaro, R, Lauro, GM, Starace, G, Fumagalli, L, (1999) "Activated alpha2 macroglobulin increase beta-amyloid (25-35) induced toxicity in LA-N-5 human neuroblastoma cells," *Exp Neuro,l,* 155(2): 252-9.

11. Beal, MF, (1995), "Aging, energy, and oxidative stress in neurodegenerative diseases, " *Ann. Neurol,* 38, 357-366.

12. Mattson, MP, (1994), "Mechanism of neuronal degeneration and preventive approaches: Quickening the pace of AD research," *Neurobiol. Ageing* 15, (Suppl.2) S121-S125.

Report on Possible Solutions in the Global Health Problems (April 2002)

-Dr. Mohamed Ahmed, M.D., President of Association of Complementary Medicine,Malaysia

The present food consumed by people in developed countries is predominantly processed food treated with pesticides, insecticides and soil nutrients of chemical nature. The introduction of many different chemicals into the body along with the food we consume has interfered with normal functioning of cells both at their intrinsic and extrinsic functions. It is now known that many proteins fold up into abnormal forms, called Rogue Proteins. These abnormal forms can be the cause of a multitude of diseases.

Example: The underlying reason why Alzheimer's and Creutzfeldt-Jakob diseases cause dementia is because small clusters of Beta Amyloid molecules—the misfolded protein—disrupt the junctions between nerve cells in rat brains. (Prof. Denis Selkoe of Harvard Medical School and colleagues.)

While scientists are trying to produce Synthetic Peptides (called Synthetic Mini-Cheperonin) to destabilize the abnormal folding of the protein, new research appears to dismiss attempts to treat the diseases by attacking the deposits and instead indicates that scientists must try to prevent the proteins misfolding in the first place.

Researchers believe that they have found the secret to correct this misfolding of proteins and sugar at the cellular level. Research in-vitro tests on neuronal cells shows that PSP+ is able to protect the neurons from toxic materials like Beta Amyloid, Peroxides and Glutamate.

Hypothesis is that PSP+ is able to provide the polysaccharide and polypeptide necessary for normal protein and sugar folding, thus enabling cellular repair.

Clinical studies in the form of *evidence based studies* prove the hypothesis. Numerous testimonials and "clinical study results" have encouraged the scientists and clinicians to indulge further into research.

With the support from the Ministry of Science and Technology of Thailand for the research projects, scientists will move even faster. More research, both in-vitro and in-vivo, is ongoing to further prove and to publish more findings. This natural food, in its simplest form, has the solution for most of the modern ailments. Instead of wasting millions of dollars on high tech surgery and medicines, we should turn to natural food, for solutions to the global problems.

Preliminary Efficacy Study of PSP+ in Multiple Sclerosis (Feb. 14 2003)[15]

-Mark Dargan Smith, N.D., PhD., Dean, University of Natural Medicine, New Mexico

Introduction

Multiple sclerosis (MS) affects 350,000 Americans. With the exception of trauma, it is the most frequent cause of neurological disability beginning in the early to middle adulthood age groups. MS is twice as common in females as in males and its occurrence is unusual before adolescence. A person has an increased risk of developing the disease from the teen years to age forty with the risk gradually declining thereafter.

MS is considered an autoimmune disease, whereby the body's own immune system (which normally targets and destroys substances foreign to the body) mistakenly attacks normal tissues. In MS, the immune system targets the brain and spinal cord, the two components of the central nervous system.

The most common symptoms of MS include:
- fatigue (most common), mental fatigue, drowsiness;
- tingling, numbness, tremors;
- sudden onset of paralysis;
- loss of balance, coordination, dizziness & lightheaded;
- weakness in one or more limbs;
- blurred or double vision; optic neuritis;
- slurred speech; swallowing problems;
- slowed thinking, decreased concentration & memory.

---

[15] The formulation used in the testing was a product labeled Vital PSP+

Methodology & Test Subjects

Three volunteers were chosen. Each was diagnosed by a physician, suffered from Multiple Sclerosis for a multitude of years and was in a very degenerative condition. The volunteers were given PSP+ to take three times daily for a period of 30-60 days.

Patient #1 & #2 had blood urine Oxidative Stress Profiles completed at days 0, 30, & 60. They filled out symptom questionnaires at days 0 & 30. It was not necessary to complete a 60-day post-test symptom questionnaire as they had few symptoms remaining at that point.

Patient #3 had a day 0 & 60 blood and urine Oxidative Stress Profile completed and also filled out the symptom questionnaires at days 0 & 60. All results are included in this clinical report. The following are the protocols that were adhered to.

Protocol

1. Test subjects met the following criteria:
   - No age limitation
   - Experiencing all of the following:
     Medical diagnosis of Multiple Sclerosis;
     The conditions or imbalances on the MS questionnaires
     (Each patient had been diagnosed with chronic degenerative Multiple Sclerosis).
13. Duration of study: 0, 30, & 60 days pre- and post-testing
14. Pre- and post testing was performed as follows:
    - Interview for qualification;
    - Physical and symptom evaluation;
    - Completed a pre and post physical and symptom assessment form;
    - Completed a MS questionnaire, before and after;
    - Pre and post Oxidative Stress Panel (blood and urine).

15. Intake (Diet, medication and supplementation).
    - Maintained: current eating habits, medications, vitamins, other supplements
    - Variable compliance on food elimination: dairy products, sugar, caffeine, alcohol and tobacco for duration of the study (optional)
16. Lifestyle
    - Maintained current lifestyle
    - Avoided long distance air travel
17. Patients completed Informed Consent Form
18. Dosage: 5 grams (1 tsp.), 3 times a day
19. The physical, symptom and laboratory measures were all completed
20. Inclusion/Exclusion criteria was followed

Laboratory Results
In one patient, who also had diabetes (type 2), self-testing indicated that there was a significant decrease in blood sugar from over 200, down to the low 100's on a consistent basis. This could be due in part to current research demonstrating that the addition of SOD (superoxide dismutase) and catalase to cultures of pancreatic islets exposed simultaneously to alloxan resulted in a partial restoration of insulin synthesis.

PSP+ delays the production of Single Molecule Sugar (Glucose). This delay will slow down the increase of the sugar in the blood, while the amino acids will help the pancreas secrete adequate insulin so sugars are brought to the cells at a more efficient rate, thereby, bringing normalcy in the blood sugar level.

The patients did not perform any internal body cleansing or detoxification procedures to enhance the elimination of toxins, which would have been the recommended protocol.

Conclusion

All three individuals participating in the study experienced significant reductions in their Multiple Sclerosis related symptoms. A reduction in degenerative disease-causing free radicals and an increase in antioxidants such as SOD (superoxide dismutase) and the glutathiones were demonstrated in the Oxidative Stress Profiles. As the SOD antioxidant increases were almost triple in the first thirty days and then declined afterward, it would most likely be attributed to the metabolism of the free radicals, a metabolic balancing, or any of the reasons previously suggested in this study.

One of the patients (with diabetes) experienced immediate and continued improvements in blood sugar regulation.

Patients experienced a normalization of weight (decrease in obesity in one, and maintaining of weight in others who did not wish to lose weight).

The results of this study along with the in-vitro research would demonstrate cellular protection from particular neurotoxins known to have a deleterious and degenerative effect on all nerve cells, (i.e. beta-amyloids, glutamates, and peroxides). The nutrients in the PSP+ would also provide the cellular fuel necessary for cellular communication and regeneration.

References

1. Laboratory report from Pacific Lab Services, Report No: /396-3971/LS 2001 Date: February 19th, 2001.
2. Mesco, ER, Timiras, PS, "Tau-ubiquitin protein conjugates I a human cell line," *Mech Ageig Dev*, 1919; 61(1): 1-9.
3. Beal, MF, (1995), "Aging, energy, and oxidative stress in neuro-degenative disease," *Ann.Neuro, 38, 357-366.*
4. Mattson, MP, (1994), "Mechanism of neuronal degeneration and preventive approaches," *Neurobiol Aging,* 15(suppl.2), S121-S125.

Glitch in Power-Generating Mitochondria Could Upset Amyloid Processing and Cellular Regeneration (March 2003)

-Dr. Bruce Yanker, M.D., Associate Professor of Neurology, Harvard Medical School

In the general population, Alzheimer's disease strikes an individual at a relatively late age, even though Mild Cognitive impairment, a potential precursor to Alzheimer's, is now found to occur at all ages. In those people with Down's syndrome the disease is more unforgiving. Most people with the syndrome develop Alzheimer's pathology by late middle age, including deposits of the plaque-forming protein amyloid-beta that are often more severe than in most other Alzheimer's patients. Why the two diseases are intimately linked is unclear. Research suggests that a malfunction in the mitochondria of Down's syndrome patients may be to blame. The resulting loss in cellular energy may explain how amyloid-beta slowly clogs the brain and why Alzheimer's is a disease of aging.

Impaired mitochondria may be to blame for the early onset of Alzheimer's disease in people with Down syndrome. This may be a result of an extra copy of chromosome 21, which can lead to the over expression of certain proteins. The amyloid precursor protein, which has beeen cleaved to form amyloid-beta, and presumably its increased production contributes to the early onset of Alzheimer's.

Specific cells with diminished mitochondrial function can accumulate the pathogenic form of amyloid-beta. A switch from the protective form to amyloid-beta could be dangerous to the cell. In culture, Down's syndrome neurons die off relatively quickly, but the team research found that a recombinant form of the protective amyloid precursor fragment could effectively rescue this degeneration.

Amyloid-beta itself comes in two sizes—the longer form is thought to be more pathogenic and toxic, and more likely to form plaque. Down's syndrome cells are in this pathogenic form, which is the direct precursor of the senile plaques. Researchers found that the trafficking of the amyloid-beta protein was also significantly altered in certain Down's syndrome cells. Normally it is quickly shuttled out of the cell once it is produced. But, in Down's syndrome cells the amyloid-beta remained inside the cell, localized in the organelles of the secretory pathway through which the precursor protein is normally trafficked. Furthermore, the protein accumulates in highly insoluble lumps.

The processing, trafficking, and folding of proteins is powered by ATP, which is generated in the mitochondria. Accumulation of amyloid beta is due to abnormal protein folding of the amyloid-beta protein once it's generated in the cells, due to loss of energy metabolism. Current findings provide a link between mitochondrial dysfunction that normally occurs in the aging brain and the predisposition to Alzheimer's. Mitochondrial dysfunction may trigger the accumulation of amyloid-beta, which impairs neurons and eventually kills them

Research has shown that feeding mitochondrial metabolites to aged rats can help slow the signs of age-related decay, suggesting a therapeutic angle on targeting the mitochondria in diseases of aging.

Authors note: PSP+ stimulates the mitochondria with the necessary metabolic fuel to not only thwart the development of the toxic amyloid-betas, but also to aid in the regeneration of new cells. This process may prevent brain cell degeneration and symptoms associated with Alzheimer's and other Neurological diseases.

Chapter Twelve

Frequently Asked Questions

Several questions in this section pertain to the supplement Vital PSP+ where results have been qualified verifying its efficacy.

Q. How are the polysaccharidepeptides in PSP different from other available polysaccharidepeptides (i.e. those found in mushrooms)?
A. The polysaccharidepeptides in PSP are the only known Alpha-Glycans, which means the structure is so small that they can be assimilated 100 percent by the body and therefore be totally absorbed into the cells. Other polysaccharidepeptides are beta-glucans, which are larger molecules and cannot be totally assimilated into the cell. Alphaglycanology assures that PSP possesses the functional characteristics that are needed in order to be recognized by the DNA and RNA.

Q. How does PSP work?
A. PSP positively influences the body by inducing an anabolic (building) phase and creating a reduction in the catabolic (breakdown) phase in order for the body to correct the metabolic disorders which are largely responsible for almost all degenerative health problems existing today. Some of the underlying symptoms of metabolic disorders include:

- free-radical attack
- Hyper-Insulinemia

- toxic colon
- hypoanabolic phase
- Metabolic Oxidative Stress
- abnormal genes
- impaired detoxification
- hypercatabolic phase
- Leaky Gut Syndrome
- Hyperlipidemia

PSP formulations are designed to enhance the body's natural healing processes by stimulating the mitochondria to produce ATP, allowing DNA repair to take place.

Q. What can the supplement Vital PSP+ do which other products cannot?
A. The best source for cellular function is a high, bioactive form of essential elements that improve the cellular environment to create a harmonious basis for ultimate gene expression. It has been proven that Vital PSP+ can work both in-vitro and in-vivo to correct degenerative health problems at the cellular level.

In-vitro studies show its efficacy in preventing injuries of neuronal cells from neurotoxins such as beta-amyloid, glutamate, and peroxides. In-vivo studies show that within ninety days, at a dosage of one measured scoop per day taken in the morning, Vital PSP+ is able to reverse the blood chemistry profile of individuals suffering from many kinds of cardiovascular and degenerative disorders. These include high cholesterol, high blood sugar, high triglycerides, high SGOT/SGPT, low in RBC, WBC and platelets counts.

Q. Is Vital PSP+ safe for pregnant or lactating women?
A. Because Vital PSP+ is a form of a whole food complex, it may provide all the basic nutrients needed by most

women. Although Vital PSP+ has not caused any problems in women who are pregnant or nursing they are asked to consult with their physician before taking Vital PSP+.

Q. Can Vital PSP+ be taken along with medications and will it interfere with the efficacy of medicines if they are taken together?
A. Reports of adverse reactions have not been forthcoming from physicians who administer Vital PSP+ together with medications. Doctors, who have had experience using Vital PSP+ along with their medication programs, including chemotherapy and radiation, have observed faster recovery from illnesses in their patients. Patients that have been on Vital PSP+ for a period of time may ask their doctor to readjust their medication, often times lessening the dosage and/or eliminating the medication entirely.

Q. Who would benefit the most from PSP?
A. Studies show daily intake of this natural whole food product can be extremely beneficial to the brain function. People who are suffering from degenerative diseases such as Alzheimer's, Multiple Sclerosis, and Parkinson's benefit the most. People suffering from arthritis, diabetes, high blood pressure, high cholesterol, strokes, attention deficit disorder and hyperactivity, and Tourette's syndrome greatly benefit from PSP.

Q. Will I go through a "healing crisis"?
A. A healing crisis is when the body's natural defense systems are waging war on the illness itself and is trying to purge the illness from the body. People whose systems are quite toxic may go through a healing crisis. During this time, symptoms may worsen. However, this healing crisis will normally only last a few short days and when over, the body heals very rapidly. Improvements in health

will be extremely noticeable. The healing crisis can be uncomfortable but once it has passed people have been astounded at how well they begin to feel. In all cases Vital PSP+ has produced positive results that have been observed in a time period ranging from a few days to as many as twelve weeks, normally averaging four to eight weeks.

Q. Can healthy people take PSP?
A. PSP is particularly valuable to individuals whose bodies are subjected to more than the usual "wear and tear." That includes those who exercise regularly, and those who are exposed to environmental stress in today's world. Modern life styles forces most people to live under stress, leaving them little or no time manage their health. Supplementing with PSP is important for our modern society even if they believe they are healthy.

Q. Is Vital PSP+ safe for pets?
A. Because Vital PSP+ is not species specific it can be given to your pets without any problem. Sprinkle a little into their food, depending on the size of the animal and encourage them to drink plenty of water. Pets will benefit in exactly the same way as humans.

Chapter Thirteen

Professional Citations[16]

If any man can convince me and bring home to me that I do not think or act aright, gladly will I change; for I search after truth, by which man never was harmed. But he is harmed who abideth on still in his deception and ignorance.
-Marcus Aurelius Antoninus

"From my own clinical observation, PSP can be safely recommended for chronically ill individuals who suffer from neurological disorders ranging from Alzheimer's, Parkinson's, Multiple Sclerosis, Meningitis, Myasthenia Gravis diseases and also stroke patients. Faster recovery was observed when PSP was given along with other forms of treatment and medications. Significant improvements in the symptoms of these patients have clearly been seen."
-Mohamed Ishak Syed Ahmad, MD, PhD, President Association of Complementary Medicine, Malaysia

"I have been using the supplement Vital PSP+ on twenty-four patients that had multiple medical problems including gastro-esophageal reflux, irritable bowel syndrome,

---

[16] The supplement Vital PSP+ was used by the professionals cited in this chapter. Therefore, their comments are specific to that product.

gastritis, and diabetes. I have been quite satisfied with the response. My patients find Vital PSP+ soothing, safe and it appeared to quiet their gut inflammation. I feel this product enhances GI healing and improves digestion from the anecdotal responses I have received."
-Norton L. Fishman, MD, Center for New Medicine, Rockville, MD

"I have been in family practice for many years. During that time I have seen many conditions benefit from a nutritional program. My first interest in nutrition began after seeing a Chronic Fatigue patient get tremendous relief from using various herbs, although I didn't know much about herbs at the time. However, due to the great results we received I started to study the wonderful means of enhancing health through nutrition. The more I read, the more I realized that even though medicine is a viable way of helping the sick, proper nutrition is a must.

Many products claim they are all natural, yet, on the label it mentions binders, fillers, and preservatives, which are far from natural. I searched for something truly all natural and after reading information on PSP I realized this was the answer for my patients various problems. I have always wanted a good nutritional product that I could recommend to my patients and their families. PSP is the perfect solution. Vital PSP+ is a great product for the whole family. We even give Vital PSP+ to our pets."
-George Michaels, DC, Los Angeles, CA

"I'm a registered nurse and have been diagnosed with chronic high blood pressure, atrial fibrillation and post-traumatic, post-operative osteoarthritis in my right knee. While I'm generally receptive to new ideas, I am usually cautious when someone introduces me to a new 'cure-all' product.

I started taking PSP on January 12, 2003. Prior to that date, I was on three blood pressure drugs (blood thinners) and potassium replacement for my cardiovascular problems. I was also taking medication for my knee pain. I was so focused on the potential cardiovascular benefits of PSP, that I didn't realize that my knee had been pain-free all week, despite the frigid cold and rainy weather. Needless to say, I stopped taking *Celebrex* and my knee remains virtually pain free.

In the meantime, I ran out of my blood pressure medications. I do not recommend that anyone stop taking any of their medications without consulting their physician and I do take my blood pressure daily. But, what I saw happening was indeed a miracle! In the past, if I needed blood pressure medication for more than two doses, I would see a dramatic increase in my pressure. Since taking PSP, in spite of not being on one of my medications, my blood pressure stays in the normal range. No combination of my prescribed medications has ever maintained a normal pressure before. I can't wait to see my cardiologist's face on my next visit. PSP may not be the cure, but I love my new PSP+ tune-up!"
-Marsha Slocum, RN, Sugar Land, TX

"PSP is the new generation of natural super foods instantly recognized by the DNA. PSP creates cellular energy that remedies an unbelievable amount of degenerative conditions, such as: Alzheimer's, MS, Cancer, AIDS, Parkinson's, Hyperactivity, Heart Disease, Diabetes, and most metabolic disorders. It is good for all ages and can improve memory function, cellular repair, blood sugar, skin conditions, hormonal function, fatigue and libido."
-J. Toan, MD, Director, Cho-ray Hospital, Vietnam

"My father, who at 81 years-old was diagnosed with fourth-stage Hepatic Cancer in mid February 2003. He had been bed and wheelchair ridden prior to and when taken to the hospital. When he was admitted he was experiencing severe pain throughout his body, especially in his bones. Upon admission, the doctors placed him on fluid therapy (electrolyte imbalance). Other symptoms he exhibited included high fever, pre-coma condition, edema and lack of energy,

The PET scan showed enlarged liver to 11x6 cm (standard size 11x11 cm). His cancer cells had migrated to the Lymphatic system. My father was told that he had only three more months to live and was released to go home because there was no further treatment available. No medication was prescribed except antipyretic drugs. But due to black color stool-bleeding the medication was stopped.

After my father was released from the hospital, I had him start taking PSP. Three weeks later the following happened: edema subsided; most of the pain disappeared; he can now walk and do normal routines; regained appetite for food; and he has much more energy. He went back to the hospital for another check-up and the doctor discovered his liver enzymes greatly improved. As a medical doctor I am a firm believer that many people can benefit by taking Vital PSP+."
-*S. Sek, MD, Bangkok, Thailand*

"As a practicing physician in the field of holistic medicine I have observed significant improvements in many patients with cognitive impairment and Parkinson's when taking PSP. In fact I would not have any reservations in recommending this product both as a preventive measure and an alternative treatment for anyone suffering from neurodegenerative disease."
-*Dr. Kampon Sriwattanakui, MD, Bangkok, Thailand*

"I have not experienced another product as effective as Vital PSP+ in remedying such a variety of illnesses and conditions. Its benefits for the entire gastro-intestinal system have been astounding. I have seen direct results in its usage for diabetes, MS, intestinal dysbiosis, gastric

ulcers and from constipation to diarrhea. PSP seems to decrease the radical damage and increase the anti-oxidants in the body."
-Mark Dargan Smith, ND, PhD, Dean of the University of Natural Medicine, Santa Fe, NM

"In my practice I use PSP to manage a variety of conditions, including Tourette's, Parkinson's, Alzheimer's, and ADD/ADHD. I advocate using whole foods instead of a multiple amount of supplements. The body can heal itself and a whole food product, such as Vital PSP+, which supports the healing process. I have noticed in myself an increase in metabolism I have lost several inches around my waist. The biggest improvement has been my eyesight. I do not have to use my glasses for distance and for reading. Cardiovascular disease and high cholesterol are very common in my family. Even though my diet is healthy and I take the various supplements that I wrote about, my cholesterol had been around 250-265. Since I began taking the product my cholesterol decreased to 215, my ratio (HDL: LDL) is 3.3 and my ratio was 5.4. All my other numbers were in the normal range. I am now in the category of a lower risk of heart attacks. Vital PSP+ is and will continue to be in my daily regimen."
-Author: Howard Peiper, ND, Albuquerque, NM

Chapter Fourteen

User Testimonials*

He that hath a truth and keeps it,
Keeps what not to him belongs.
But performs a selfish action,
And a fellow mortal wrongs.
—Andrew Jackson Davis

*The supplement Vital PSP+ was used by the people who are cited in this chapter. Their results are specific to that product.

Conditions treated within this chapter:

Back Pain	Goiter
Blood Pressure	Hip problems
Cancer	Hyperactivity
Carpal Tunnel	Hypertension
Cerebral Palsy	Leg Pain
Chronic Fatigue	Lupus
Colitis	Migraines
Diabetes	Overweight conditions
Eczema	Parkinson's
Flu	Seizures
Fibromyalgia	Stroke
Gangrene	Tourette's

Back Pain

"A severe whiplash from a car accident eight years ago gave me chronic neck and lower back pain. Consequently, I have suffered from lower-space-disc disease and have found that just lifting five to ten pounds is very difficult. After taking PSP three times a day for only one week, I could pick up my two and one-half year-old grandson, who weighs thirty pounds, without any pain. Before PSP I felt like I was old. I am so excited, I am telling everyone!"
-Hilarie Crone, York, PA

Blood Pressure

"My husband blood pressure fluctuated between 160/98 and 170/102 for four and one-half years. He was on *Accupril*, at a dosage of 10mg a day. He started taking PSP on January 13th along with his *Accupril*. After one week, he discontinued the *Accupril*. Since I am in the medical field, I could monitor Mike and took his blood pressure twice a day. His blood pressure was running 140/90–150/92, safe enough to continue to monitor without using the *Accupril*.

After three and one-half weeks he went off the medication and his blood pressure ran 128/78-140/82. He is taking PSP only once in the morning and he is feeling great. I will continue to monitor his blood pressure. The only change in his lifestyle is the PSP and since using it we have seen a major improvement."
-Rita Wynegar, York, PA

Blood Pressure

"Four years ago I was diagnosed with high blood pressure. My doctor had me on four medications. Even with these medications my blood pressure sometimes reached 180/100. I have lived in fear of a heart attack during recent years. I was introduced to PSP during the first week in December 2002. I began a protocol of taking one scoop

three times a day. On January 1, 2003, I checked my blood pressure and was shocked to find that it was 126/64. This is considered a low reading for me. My doctor has now reduced the dosage of all my medications. One day I know I will be able to eliminate them. Praise the Lord for PSP. I now have a future to look forward to."
-John Doak, El Paso, TX

High blood pressure
"High blood pressure runs in my family "My blood pressure in September 2002 was 144/90. I have only been taking PSP since January 2003 at two doses a day, and my blood pressure has dropped to 128/73. This improvement is very encouraging to me.

Meanwhile, my husband had open-heart surgery in January 2003. Postoperative blood work revealed that he had high cholesterol, high blood pressure and high triglycerides. The doctor advised him to get his counts down immediately or he would be right back in the hospital with more blockage problems. I started him on PSP as an adjunct to his regular medications and gave our family physician information on the product.

After 1½ months of him being on PSP three times daily, I was anxious to have his blood work redone. The results subsequently revealed that all his counts were either significantly lowered or within normal limits: Cholesterol went from 244 to 127; Triglycerides from 471 to 221; and the Chol/HDL ratio from 6.10 to 5.08. His blood pressure is also down to normal. Well, needless to say, our family doctor was quite surprised and even shocked with the results after such a short time. He asked us for additional information on PSP. Under his doctor's supervision, I am now working towards weaning my husband totally off his medications."
-Betty Atland, York, PA

Colon Cancer

"In August 2001 I was diagnosed with colon cancer. I had an operation and was put on chemotherapy treatments. Later on, I was diagnosed with Parkinson's disease and suffered from tremors, dizziness and chronic fatigue. In May 2002 I started taking PSP and over the course of about one year I observed fewer problems with my tremors. The symptoms of dizziness and chronic fatigue have disappeared. My immune system is back to a healthy state, even after having chemotherapy."
-Phrakru Tien (Thai Monk), Bangkok, Thailand

Carpal Tunnel

"My name is Morrie Louden. I've been a professional Bassist (Musician) for thirty years. I got carpal tunnel syndrome about four years ago from having to play my standup bass six days a week. It was serious enough to have surgery. The surgery improved the situation a bit, but the pain was still there. I began using PSP. After the first week, the pain had subsided. Five weeks later I realized I was now capable of working steady and have gone back to playing six days a week without a bit of pain. WOW! I wish I'd have known sooner about PSP. It would have prevented my surgery!"
-Morrie Louden, Austin, TX

Cerebral Palsy

"Fatin was born in 1995 and was diagnosed with Cerebral Palsy. Since birth, she has suffered from stunted growth, physical weakness and was always sick. With so many neurological deficiencies she was very difficult to manage. We tried everything from medicines to herbs and various forms of supplements, but we saw no improvement in her condition.

In October 2000 when Fatin was five and one half years old, we started to give her PSP and noticed rapid improvement with her neurological functions. She started

to sit and stand (with some assistance), something she was not able to do before. She became more alert, started to understand what was being said to her, and was more responsive. Nowadays, she seldom gets colds, flu, or fever. As of February 2002 Fatin has grown stronger and her interactions with others have been miraculous. We will continue to give her Vital PSP+."
-Shamsuddin Malik, Fatin's father, Johore, Malaysia

Chronic Fatigue
"I have been suffering from Chronic Fatigue Syndrome for many years. My naturopathic doctor suggested that I start taking a unique whole food formula from Thailand. He had learned that this amazing whole food was helping others who had various immune-suppression ailments. Since taking Vital PSP+, my energy level has gotten much better. My aches and pains are gone and my immune system is stronger."
-Marge Smith, Albuquerque, NM

Colitis & Rosacea
" My wife, Joan, has had colitis for the last six months, and has also had a serious asthmatic condition for several years. In January, I put her on PSP. After just one month, she has been able to eliminate her colitis medicine completely. She has also reduced her inhaler use by 50 percent. She has resumed activities such as shoveling her car out of the snow by herself, and sledding with her thirteen-year-old grandson. Without the PSP, this would have been unheard of. Due to her testimony, I started taking the product. I've noticed that my energy has increased and the rosacea on my face, which has been steadily getting worse for the past year, has receded by 70 percent. There is no doubt to the efficacy of PSP."
-John Throne, York, PA

Diabetes

"I was diagnosed with Type II Diabetes in 1998. I am a very large lady and have had poor results with many diabetic prescriptions. My blood sugar was 160 when, on January 15, 2003 I started taking PSP. After two days my blood sugar dropped to 140—a miracle! On January 17th, only four days after starting PSP, my blood sugar was 118! This is nothing short of awesome!"
-Beverly Peasley, Elizabethtown, KY

Dialysis patient

"I have been a dialysis patient for three years and am currently undergoing the procedure three times per week. Ever since I started the dialysis, my skin turned dark, I lost my energy, and I felt constantly fatigued. I had to rest for an hour after being on the dialysis machine. My feet were swollen and numb from retaining fluids causing me many sleepless nights.

After taking PSP for only two months, I noticed the following changes: my skin went back to its original color; I could do housework without feeling fatigued; and I was able to get up and walk immediately after each dialysis. I now sleep well through the night and I am certain that by taking PSP, my dialysis frequency will someday be reduced."
-Lee Sen, Melaka, Malaysia

Eczema

"Since her birth, my daughter, Mei Jin, had never had a restful day or even a restful night due to itchy lesions. After she had been on PSP for nine weeks, I noticed that 80-90 percent of her eczema lesions slowly had disappeared. I thank the people who introduced to me Vital PSP+. I no longer use any more antibiotics or steroids on Mei Jin's skin."
-Lim Mei Jin, Mei Jin's mother, Singapore

Flu

"My twelve-year-old son came home with a miserable headache and his whole body hurt (typical flu-like symptoms). I immediately gave him some *Tylenol* for the pain but it did not work. He was up all night with a terrible headache, body ache and a slight fever. The next morning I realized that we should try the PSP. I gave him a dose with some warm tea at 8:30 A.M. and by 9:00 A.M., his fever was virtually gone and his headache and body aches were also eliminated. This is so amazing! He told me how much better he had felt. I attribute his quick recovery to the PSP. All I have to say is, wow! Children can totally benefit from taking PSP."
-Tania DeQuattro, Columbia, SC

Fibromyalgia and colds

"I use PSP for my fibromyalgia and irritable-bowel syndrome. I was so pleased with how I felt that I decided to give my son a half scoop of Vital PSP every day. He had been suffering constantly from a runny and a stuffy nose. Now he no longer suffers. If he does get a cold, he only gets a runny nose if I forget to give him Vital PSP+ a few days in a row."
-Sherry Adams, AZ

Gangrene

"I have suffered with Diabetes for eleven years. I now also have Neuropathy, Retinopathy and Nephropathy. Because of a sore on my right ankle I developed an ulcer that turned into gangrene. My wound was not responding to medication and the doctors suggested amputation (below my knee). I started taking PSP three times a day along with ozone treatment. I also applied PSP locally to my wound. My diet has been controlled through eating high protein foods and eliminating carbohydrates. I eventually got off my insulin. Within a short period of time, all edema around the wound settled down and I was able to

walk short distances. My doctor had me finish taking a course of antibiotics and stated that my wound was healing extremely well. When I returned for the next appointment, a skin grafting was scheduled. Thanks to PSP, I can now play basketball and jog. What a gift!"
-*Mohamed Zain, Prof. of Engineering, University Tech of Malaysia*

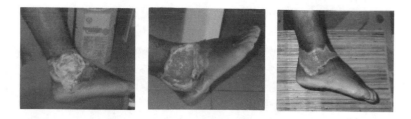

September 18. 2001   September 26, 2002   October 29, 2002

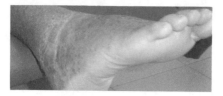

February 18, 2003
Gangrene healed

Goiter

"I have suffered from abnormal thyroid function for the past seventeen years and have had a goiter on my neck for this entire period. Doctors advised me to have an operation and for some reason I refused. PSP was introduced to me and within three months my goiter greatly reduced its size. Now it is just about gone. I am glad my intuition told me that there was an alternative to surgery."
-*Tak Koh, Singapore*

Hip Replacement

"I started taking the PSP product in February, 2003, in preparation for a total hip replacement that was to take place in April. I had the surgery and was discharged three days later a day earlier than expected (usually patients that have had total hip replacements must stay for four or five days after surgery). Two weeks after discharge from the hospital I started taking the PSP product every day. In only a few weeks, I could easily go up and down stairs and walk over a mile just for fun. My physical therapist report read 'doing extremely well.'

The therapist told me that my recovery would most likely be 40 percent faster than the typical hip replacement patient—which means 40 percent less expensive to me. I'm 59 years old, and have invested my professional life in being a health care economist and medical practice consultant. Taking PSP as been the best health care investment I've ever made. I believe the PSP product could have significant benefits towards lowering health care costs."

-Clifford Todd, Newport Beach, CA

Hip Dysplasia in a dog.

"I ordered Vital PSP+ for my husband who is diabetic and who is getting remarkable results. So I thought about giving Vital PSP+ to my eight year old German Shepard, Heidi who has hip dysplasia. In about one week I noticed she was moving better. She was going up the stairs without help or making sure someone was behind her when she did. She also has more energy. I just put about a quarter of a scoop of Vital PSP+ in her food once a day."

-Candella Shaffer, Dallas, TX

Hyperactivity

"My seven year-old son Jesus, has had hyperactivity problems since he was three years old. Jesus was very easily distracted, unable to count to more than forty and to

67

maintain concentration on any subject. Most of the time, I couldn't put him to sleep. He used to watch TV until one o'clock in the morning.

After about a month of taking PSP, we noticed Jesus was able to count up to four hundred or more without losing concentration. He can count by fives up to two hundred sixty. His teacher told us that he is now one of the most behaved students in the class. He now goes to sleep at 8:00 P.M."
-Anna Dominguez, Soledad, CA

Hypertension, hyperthyroidism
"I've suffered from hypertension, hyperthyroidism and have been overweight for about thirteen years. Because of poor night vision, my driving has always been bad while driving at night. Since taking PSP, my vision has improved and I've also lost fifteen pounds. My doctor told me that my blood pressure and my thyroid are now normal. I don't take hypertension and hyperthyroid medication anymore. These improvements were observed only after a few months on PSP, taking it three times a day."
-Dodi Cruz, Bellwood, IL

Leg Pain and Diabetes
"I have experienced severe pain in my left leg since I had back surgery in 1991. My doctors told me I had irreversible nerve damage. This was unwelcome news to anyone, but especially for a person who had insulin-dependent diabetes. The pain made it very difficult to walk. Two weeks after I started taking PSP, the pain subsided enough that I stopped taking pain pills. My doctor was amazed. Since taking PSP, I have been able to reduce my insulin from 32 units a day to 18 units. "
-George Stein, NY

Leg pain

"I am a building inspection supervisor for a mid-sized city and have suffered with a pain that shoots up my leg and causes me to limp. Over-the-counter pain medications do not help. I started taking PSP on January 13, 2003. After only four days on this product, I realized that I was not limping. Another benefit I received is that I simply felt better!"

-Darrel "Hap" Watkins, Portland, OR

Lupus

"My name is Tammy Bennett and I have SLE (Systemic Lupus Erythmatosus), Sjoren's disease and anemia. Most people have never heard of Lupus and those that have, usually don't understand the disease. (Our bodies make too many white blood cells. These cells then lose the ability to distinguish between the body and invading organisms. As a result, the body starts attacking itself.) The symptoms vary and while some people don't even know that they have the disease or have a very mild case, others die from complications of lupus. Fatigue is a very common symptom. Lupus symptoms I have had include mouth ulcers, weight gain (70 pounds), hair loss, anxiety, mood changes, depression, muscle weakness, headaches and constant pain. Last year was particularly difficult because of an onset of severe depression.

In January 2003 my best friend called with some news of a whole food complex that was supposed to help with the symptoms of lupus. I was very skeptical but I agreed to talk to my rheumatologist about it. My doctor stated he was not familiar with the ingredients in PSP+, however, he didn't think it would hurt for me try it for ninety days. Since taking PSP, that I have noticed more energy, and that in general, I feel better physically and emotionally.

PSP is not just changing my life; it is giving me my life back. My doctor and I are looking forward to comparing my last test results with the next blood test."
-Tammy Bennett, Tampa, Fl.

Migraines

"I have been suffering from migraine headaches for the past seven years, usually at a rate of one per month. They were so severe I wasn't able to do very much for three days. I have been taking PSP for a little over three months and have not had one migraine headache. It is great to not losing those three days a month I can now be productive."
-Kathy Shunkwiler, Hallam, NE

Multiple Sclerosis

"I have had Multiple Sclerosis and elevated blood sugar problems for many years. I am wheel chair bound. In 1986 I experienced weakness in my hands and I was hospitalized with a blood sugar crisis. I was in the VA hospital for a month. I have quadriplegia, greater in my legs and on my left side. I have lost more than two-thirds of my muscle strength. My SOD (antioxidant) level was 1,542, which was below standard.

Only thirty days after I started taking a food supplement called PSP, my SOD level went up to 3,158 and I can tell you that now my feet are much healthier. They are not as red or swollen as they used to be and are looking normal. I had stiffness, mostly in my left ankle and knee— now I am more mobile. My thighs also are not as stiff and I notice I am developing more muscle on them. The strength in my arms and legs has improved. I used to let my care provider push me all the time in my wheel chair when we were out, but now I push myself most of the time.

I went to the barbershop a few days ago and for the first time I could get off the electric scooter and into the barber chair by myself. Before, two men had to help

me up. I have also lost quite a few pounds during this short time. I am very grateful to Vital PSP+ for turning my life around."
-Francisco Gabaldon, Santa Fe, NM

Multiple Sclerosis

"For many years, I suffered with "MS brain fog" and had to work hard to think well. I could not decide if it was from MS (Multiple Sclerosis) or the beginning of a senile dementia. The severe headaches continued off and on and MS fatigue continued. I had too little energy to even consider walking around a large grocery store. It was customary for me to be in bed eleven to twelve hours a night and not awaken refreshed. My SOD (antioxidant) level was 1,728.

Thirty days after I started to take PSP on a daily basis, I felt considerably better. My SOD level had doubled to 3,766. Each day I recognized significant improvement. I no longer wear an ankle brace for support, something that I had done for years. I have not had any spasticity in my legs and back since taking PSP+. Also, the edema in my legs is markedly less and they look nearly normal. Other changes I had observed included greater bladder control as well as a reduction in my medication (Synthroid) that was prescribed for a hypothyroid condition.

I now can do physical things that I could not do during past years. The oppressive multiple sclerosis fatigue is nearly gone. My support group said at this month's meeting that I looked years younger and I was walking very well. I am thrilled at the return of near normal health and look expectantly each day for new improvements."
-Janice South, Santa Fe, NM

Overweight and allergic

"I used to weigh 250 pounds and have suffered from a stuffy nose and skin allergies for many years. I could not work long hours due to fatigue and tiredness. After one month of taking PSP, my vitality has come back. I don't tire as easily as I used to. I can now work longer hours and even my bowel movements have greatly improved."
-Maria Dominguez, Soledad, CA

Parkinson's

"I have had a serious problem with Parkinson's disease. The last six months I have not been sleeping very well. Even after taking sleeping pills, I could not sleep very long, sleeping just two to three hours at a time. I was introduced to PSP in March of 2002. The first week I only took the PSP one time a day. Then I started taking PSP three times a day and began getting great results. I now sleep without any sleeping pills for six to eight hours. I feel rested and energetic when I wake up in the morning. My friends that know me are amazed at how well I look."
-Jose Zuniga, Tijuana, Mexico

Rosacea and spastic muscle control

"Ryan is seventeen years old and was born with a spastic right arm and leg. His limbs worked, but the fine motor skills were poor. Ryan began taking PSP on January 12, 2003 in a dosage of twice per day. After one week, Ryan came to me and showed me the movement in his right wrist. He has always only been able to move his hand at the wrist up and down; movement left and right could only be achieved by force. He was now able to move his wrist freely in *all* directions. I also noticed that when he ran across the floor at a basketball game (ten days after being on the PSP) that he ran much more normal. His right arm didn't come up like it used to. His complexion has cleared up (and for a teenager, this is a major priority)

and he hasn't been complaining about his allergies. I don't have to remind him to take the PSP as he is seeing results and is determined to eventually have full use of his right arm. By the way, the medications that Ryan has been on are slowly being eliminated."
-*Deb Bunn, Ryan's Mom, Des Moines IA*

Author's note: *When I met Ryan's mom and told her that Vital PSP+ could help him with his ailments, she had tears in her eyes. I believe and they believed.*

Rosacea

"I went to see my mother who is forty-nine years old and suffers from Rosacea, which is also known as adult acne. Rosacea affects 14 million Americans today and can be treated but not cured. It causes facial swelling and redness with visible signs of blood vessels. She has been fighting Rosacea for several years. I gave her the PSP and within one week the Rosacea was barely noticeable. She is only taking one scoop a day. We can't wait to see what the next thirty days will bring."
-*Casey Minshew, Houston, TX*

Stroke

"On January 11, 2003 I was introduced to PSP and it has changed my life! Five years ago a blood clot traveled to my brain and caused a stroke. After eighteen months of speech, physical and occupational therapy, I was showing little progress and I no longer qualified for services. All therapy was stopped.

The left side of my body was affected from the stroke as was my speech and ability to walk. I have had very little use of my left arm, and my left hand had re-mained in a fist position. I have always been a lefty and by not having the use of the left hand I have had to deal with a big adjustment. I was always tired and needed to sleep a lot. I never felt energized.

I started taking PSP on the evening of January 11 in the amount of three times a day. Several wonderful things happened. My left arm was no longer contracted—it was hanging down by my side in a relaxed, natural position (this is the arm that has not been straight in years). I could voluntarily open and close my left hand and I could even hold a deodorant bottle in my left hand! My speech and my thinking both were notably clearer. I now sleep very well at night and actually look forward to getting up, in fact, I am up to thirty sit-ups every morning! I still take an afternoon nap, but I do not require the sleep I did before I started taking PSP+.

Other people are noticing the difference in me. They cannot always pinpoint what is different; they just say I looked great! I had only been on this product sixteen days and I knew firsthand what it could do. I am my own testimonial. Thank you for Vital PSP+. The last two weeks have been so remarkable. I am truly looking forward to the months ahead. Who knows what the total outcome will be?"
–Jim Nicholson, Maynard, IA

Stroke

"My wife, Neyda, is sixty-eight years old, and suffered a severe stroke in July 2001. She was in a coma for more than eighteen days. The doctors predicted that she would be bed- and wheelchair-bound for the rest of her life. The left side of her body was paralyzed. She could not express herself nor recognize her family. She had to be helped with all her needs including eating.

In the spring of 2002, she started taking PSP three times a day. After only six weeks, she was able to stand and take steps. She had movement and control over her left side of her body. She had started to exercise and take physical therapy. She also began to lift a weight of one pound with her left leg and arm, both of which had been previously paralyzed.

I had witnessed her progress with my own eyes every time I visited her. Her doctors and relatives were amazed with her progress. The prognosis is favorable that she may recover almost completely from her stroke."
-*Jose Matos, San Juan. PR*

Tourette's syndrome

"Haley, my nine-year old daughter, was diagnosed this summer with Tourette's, a condition that causes uncontrolled muscle movements. Haley's tics were mainly facial. She'd also gasp for air when she was very excited or upset. Drugs are prescribed for Tourette's but because of their terrible side effects we decided against them.

ADHD (attention deficit hyperactivity disorder) is associated with Tourette's, and Haley was also experiencing trouble concentrating in school and at home. When she was frustrated with herself, the tics would worsen.

I was introduced to PSP and hoped this was the answer to my prayers. I started her on one dose a day in the morning and within four days her dad and I both noticed her tics were gone! We just couldn't believe it happened so quickly. Therefore, we assumed it was just a fluke. Then after a week and still no tics, we started believing it was the PSP. We asked Haley if she felt different and she said yes. She explained she was having an easier time concentrating at school and other kids didn't distract her as easily as before. We are noticing she minds better at home and doesn't forget things at school as she previously had done.

Her tics came back during one period in her recovery and we discovered the reason; she wasn't taking all of her Vital PSP+ in the morning! Now we are closely monitoring her to make sure she gets the full dosage. When she follows the recommended dosage her tics go

away. I can't thank the people enough who introduced Vital PSP+ to me. It has truly changed Haley's life and ours as well."
-*Linda Lutz, Haley's mom, Minneapolis, MN*

Author's note: *I have written two best sellers on ADD/ADHD and have found that over 50 percent of the children that are on Ritalin for hyperactivity actually have Tourette's. Ritalin aggravates Tourette's syndrome.*

Conclusion

*Let no one presume to give advice to others that has
not first given good advice to himself.*
—Seneca

The information and statistics from the previous chapters will mean nothing to you unless you take action. This is more than a book about PSP. It is a book about people like you—individuals who are in search of health and natural healing. The people who told their personal stories all felt that PSP had changed their lives. For some, it was miraculous, and for others it was significant enough to make the quality of their lives much better. PSP is a product unlike any other. You deserve the best quality of life, health, and wellness and PSP can restore and preserve that health for a lifetime.

Resources

Vital PSP+ is available from quality nutritional representatives of Healthywize products. For information and products, contact the nutritional representative who gave you this book or contact the company at:
(866) PSP-5050 (777-5050).

INDEX

Bibliography

-Anderson, Nina, Peiper, Howard *Secrets of Staying Young*, Safe Goods Publishing, 1999.
-Bell, Rachel, Peiper, Howard, *The ADD & ADHD Diet*, Safe Goods Publishing, 2001.
-Ishak, Dr. Mohammed, "Possible Solutions to the Global Health Problems, " *Nature's Journal*, April 2002.
-Khalsa, Dharma, *Brain Longevity*, Warner Books, 1999.
-Page, Linda, *Healthy Healing, 11th Edition*, Traditional Wisdom, 2000.
-Natures Journal #444, p. 632-636, 2001.
-Humphries, Courtney, "Glitch in Power-generating Mitochondria could upset Amyloid Processing and Cellular Regeneration," *Harvard Research*, Feb 2003.
-"Healing Hepatitis Naturally," *Dr. Rx for Healthy Living*, Freedom Press, 2000.
-Peiper, Howard, *Naturopathic Secrets of Your pH*, Natures Publishing, 2002.
-Wise, SJ, *The Sugar Addict's Diet*, Safe Goods Publishing, 2000.

Other Books available through ATN Publishing

Nutritional Leverage for Great Golf Improving your score on the back nine	$ 9.95
The Backseat Flyer A passenger's guide to flying	$ 9.95
Eliminating Pilot Error The final step in flight training	$ 7.95
2012 Airborne Prophesy An environmental conspiracy novel	$16.95
Spirit & Creator The Man behind Lindbergh's Flight to Paris	$39.95

Titles by Dr. Howard Peiper

The Secrets of Staying Young	$ 9.95
High Performance Diet	$ 7.95
ADD, The Natural Approach	$ 4.95
The ADD & ADHD Diet	$ 9.95
Natural Solutions for Sexual Enhancement	$ 9.95
Super Nutrition for Dogs n' Cats	$ 9.95
All Natural Anti-Aging Skin Care	$ 4.95
Recharge Your Biological Battery	$ 6.95
Nutritional Leverage for Great Golf	$ 9.95

For a complete listing of books by ATN Publishing
and Safe Goods Publishing visit our web site:
www.safegoodspub.com or call for a free catalog
(888) NATURE-1 (628-8731)

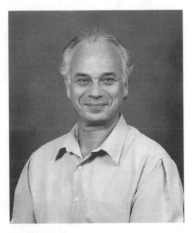

Author

Dr. Howard Peiper, N.D.

Dr. Howard Peiper N.D., nominated for a Pulitzer Prize has written/co-authored many books on nutrition and natural health including the best-seller, *The A.D.D. and A.D.H.D. Diet.*